30 Intentions
in
30 Days

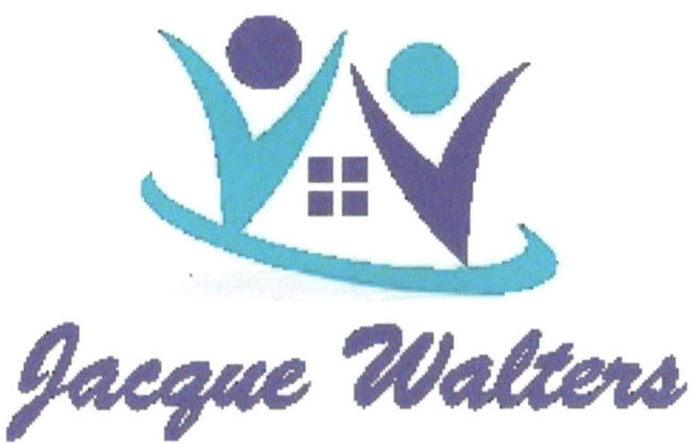

Disclaimer

Not all exercise movements are suitable for everyone. To reduce the risk of injury, consult your doctor before beginning any exercises suggested in this book. The information in this book and the accompanying videos are not medical advice. This information is intended for educational purposes only and not to be used to self-diagnose or self-treat any medical condition. If you experience any pain or difficulty while doing any of the suggested intentions, stop immediately and see your healthcare professional.

Copyright © 2018 Jacque Walters

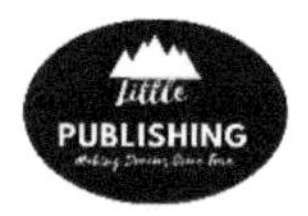

DEDICATION

I dedicate this book to anyone in physical pain wanting to find
a way to heal naturally.

ACKNOWLEDGMENTS

I would like to thank all the clients and students I have had throughout my fitness career. You are the reason I love this professional path and journey. Your support and confidence helped motivate me to keep learning and growing to serve you to the very best of my abilities.

I would also like to acknowledge my mentor, Virginia Parsons for her unending faith and belief in me to keep stepping outside the box, face my fears and just go for it. Thank you from the bottom of my heart. AND thank you for being my "high tech guru" with my website and videos.

I want to thank, Danae C Little for seeing something in me that I would never have known. Being a writer and publishing a book was the furthest thing from my mind. Your support has been amazing, and I am so grateful for all your help including being my editor and publisher.

Finally, I would like to thank Patrick Mummy who worked tirelessly to create "SYMMETRY." He not only helped thousands of individuals personally but created a system so that those he trained and certified could teach this amazing program to help many thousands more.

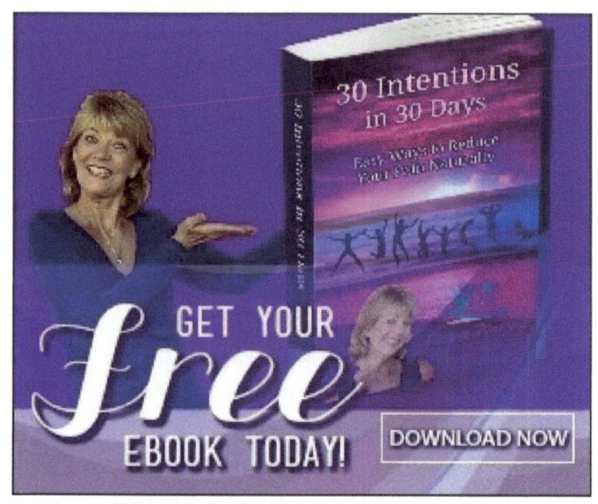

Here is a **FREE** digital version of this book with **clickable links** to videos and information!

www.jacquewalters.com/30-intention/

You can also download my FREE GUIDE,
4 Easy Movements
at:

www.jacquewalters.com/4emoptin/

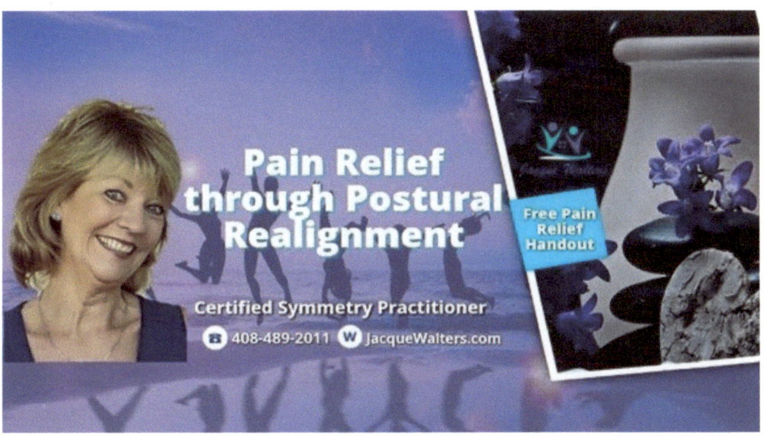

INTRODUCTION

You are the reason I wrote this book. I believe in you! YOU have the power within you to reduce and even eliminate pain. I believe in your body's ability to heal if given the chance. I believe in you because only YOU can go within, allow yourself to open up, learn how to heal, and practice what you are taught. That's when the magic happens—naturally.

Do you want to reduce pain naturally without drugs or surgery? If your answer is yes, read on.

One of my clients had undergone back surgery and was still having pain issues. She told me she wished she would have met me prior to the procedure. She had believed the surgery would take her pain away. Unfortunately, it made things worse. My response was to encourage her to start from right now and begin a new journey. It is never too late.

I repeat—IT IS NEVER TOO LATE!!!!!!!!

This book is not just about offering **4 Easy Movements** to begin the journey to reduce pain, but to also pass on "fit tips" that do not take hours to do and yet produce amazing results. If your life is busy and spending hours in the gym is challenging, then these suggestions are for you.

I have spent the last 25 years of my 45+ years in the fitness industry researching and finding ways to get the greatest results in the least amount of time with the least amount of effort. Because here is the thing: **I am probably the laziest fitness professional in the industry.**

Really, I am. I don't like to spend much time working out. However, I want to be healthy, strong and stay at my ideal weight throughout my senior years. Oh, did I mention I am a senior citizen? I also had chronic pain for years from an accident and I am now pain free.

I am not in pain because I faithfully do what I teach. Everything in this book is what I do personally. I incorporate these ideas into my days throughout the week. Some intentions I do daily, like my gratitude walk with my dog, Molly. I also eat a clean diet and do "mindful" daily practices.

I am not here to convince you to stop doing your favorite form of exercise. There are so many wonderful choices within the industry and there is a therapeutic effect when working out with others. Many fitness experts claim to have the best way to become fit, so it can be confusing if you haven't found your favorite. Don't give up, keep looking and asking. The referral system is the best way to find a fitness professional you can resonate with.

So, if you have a favorite, keep doing it. However, if you are in pain with what you are doing then something needs to change. Going to the gym a few times a week for an hour workout does not counteract hours upon hours of chronic uninterrupted sitting. You need to consistently exert your body against gravity. Only frequent upright movement will do that. Meaning, you want to interrupt your sitting as often as possible. That is what the intentions in this book are all about. As I said earlier, I wrote it just for you.

When I tell my friends and clients that I am writing a book about setting small intentions and admit I that I am lazy, they all look at me as though I am crazy. They are actually shocked that I see myself as lazy. My clients give me all kinds of examples of what I do.

One of my secrets is that I don't set huge expectations with my workout intentions. (I like the word "intentions" better than goals or resolutions.) Then I just pick one and do it. I find that once I get going, I go beyond what I first intended, AND I only spend as little as 3 to 5 minutes. I do several of my mini workouts throughout the day.

Making huge resolutions may work for some people, but not for me. So, I ask you: Do you set your intentions (goals) so high that they are unattainable? Then do you feel horrible when you don't achieve them and end up feeling like a failure? Do you feel guilty when you miss a workout or fitness class? Try one of my mini workouts to make up for it on one those busy days or "I don't feel like it" days so you don't have to feel bad. I DON'T EVER WANT YOU TO FEEL BAD! That is another reason this book is for YOU.

I am very happy with my way of doing things and it works for me. You need to discover what "really" works for you.

Studies have been conducted that are revealing that short bursts of exercise are actually just as beneficial as longer workouts. How does it get any better that that? Less time working out with the same results—I love it!

I would like to share some of those studies with you now. Click on the link below to get started.
http://journals.plos.org/plosone/article?id=10.1371/journal.pone.0154075

Here are more studies about shorter workouts rather than longer ones. The results from the shorter workouts can be even more beneficial with regards to arterial pliability and blood pressure spikes.
https://well.blogs.nytimes.com/2013/07/05/ask-well-3-short-workouts-or-1-long-one/

The research in this article is about the effects of mortality rates with a sedentary lifestyle.
http://www.thelancet.com/journals/lancet/article/PIIS0140-6736(16)30370-1/fulltext

Just start with getting up and moving more and see what happens. Don't get wrapped up in big ideas or set huge goals. Start small, and then go a little further and exceed beyond what you first set out to accomplish.

My suggestions can help you with starting small. Baby step intentions can turn out to be way more advantageous than unattainable goals.

Remember to also fidget and move a lot when you are sitting, shifting and changing your position often. And of course, get up frequently and move. Which is what this book is about.

Am I repeating myself? I hope so.

This book is not only about giving you suggested "**Intentions**" but also for journaling your answers to questions I pose and other thoughts that come to mind. Here's a question: Have you ever thought about all the benefits of journaling? Below is a website stating 10 benefits of journaling along with links to the research. It can even boost your immune system! Wow!
https://www.huffingtonpost.com/thai-nguyen/benefits-of-journaling-b_6648884.html

How about giving it a try by answering the following questions?

Did you check out the research? If so, what were your thoughts about it?
____

____

____

____

Are any of these ideas new to you?
____

So, what do you have to lose besides a longer, healthier life free of pain and discomfort?
____

____

____

I worded the question that way purposely to shake up your thought process. Did it work?
____

Let me rephrase it. Do you want to live a longer healthier life free of pain and discomfort? There, better? _______________________________________

What would that look like for you?
____

____

____

____

____

____

____

____

____

____

Before moving on to the <u>30 Intentions in 30 Days</u>, I want to talk about the **4 Easy Movements.** It is not just about the exercises themselves. They are basic, and you have probably seen or done them before. It is the "how and why" they are done in the order given that is the magic.

THE HOW AND WHY

The response to my <u>4 Easy Movements to Relieve Pain Naturally</u> has been very exciting. I am thrilled that this free gift that only takes minutes allows an individual to begin to feel the changes taking place. Read on and I will explain the how and why.

Why do individuals get relief from even the first easy movement?

The Symmetry Program is a physics-based program. It is all about gravity, gravitation, and Newton's third law. "For every action there is an equal and opposite reaction." The first movement is actually a non-movement.

Postural re-alignment is about reprogramming both your brain and body. It takes thousands of repetitions to undo faulty muscle fiber recruitment patterns. Most adults have had years of dysfunctional patterning. Postural therapy is reeducating the neurological system, so the entire body is able to stand in an optimal upright position with the left and right sides mirroring each other. That system includes the brain. So, the communication and neural pathways between the brain and the muscles of the body both need reprogramming. "The neuromuscular process to getting to the walking stage is a long but intentional path that allows us to get to our natural design – which is to stand on two feet and to move." (Symmetry Core Level One Training 2014)

In other words, your body was hard wired before you were even born to develop in certain sequences and patterns. Your first year of life was all about being on your back and then rolling over to pushing up (babies automatically know the cobra position). Then you moved to sitting, falling over many times in the learning process, but you never gave up. You then automatically went on your hands and knees and rocked until crawling began. You finally pulled yourself to stand in an optimal postural stance and took those first steps.

Then once upright on two feet, the human body just keeps moving—not only walking, but running. Little ones never stop moving from the time of conception. We are programmed and built to keep moving. Yet all the conveniences in our high-tech world now have us <u>sitting too much</u>. This problem is having a huge impact on our health.

Movement #1: Gravity is your friend to help with the process.

Subtle corrections begin to happen when doing the first (non) movement. More than 90% of your brain's output is to maintain your body in the gravitational field. So, the first thing that happens is the brain is able to rest from this output because you are being fully supported. All load bearing joints (ankles, knees, hips and shoulders) need to rest and lie side by side with no effort so the neurological reprogramming can begin.

Offsets in your spine will begin to change back toward better alignment as you relax. Your knees and feet will be let go of tightness and fatigue. Your pelvis begins to let go of the tension that is created because it is the base of locomotive power in your body. Your shoulders begin to settle and open up. This position allows your brain to begin the important reprogramming process.

There are 1440 minutes in a 24-hour period. This first exercise in the **4 Easy Movements** takes only 3 to 5 minutes.

Do you believe you are worth at least 3 minutes to begin healing naturally?

Movement #2: Next we address the shoulders.

This 2nd free exercise is designed to help undo deviations in the shoulder girdle, specifically shoulder elevation. The head always wants to be directly over the center of gravity in the body. When there are misalignments in the hips or shoulders, the head will automatically move to the center resulting in offsets in the spine. These offsets upset the natural curvature of the spine and in many cases leads to pain somewhere in the neck, mid back, or low back, as well as, shoulder discomfort and hip pain.

Many muscles are involved with the 2nd movement of this exercise. These include chest, back, and shoulder muscles. They are all important in the corrective action. The wonderful result of this 2nd movement is the shoulders (which are made up of 4 joints) begin to move toward a level position when you are once again standing upright.

The exercise is so simple yet give remarkable results. It is important to repeat the movement pattern at least 20 times. Then after a couple of deep breaths, the repetitions are repeated. First the brain and neurological pathways begin to be reprogrammed symmetrically. Then a second set is done to continue the reprogramming within the muscles. This exercise only takes a little over a minute. How easy is that?

Movement #3: It is time to talk about the hips.

The hip joint is one of the most strong, secure, and stable joints in the body. This stability is due to its boney structure and the powerful muscles surrounding the joint; and a strong, fibrous capsule reinforced by ligaments.

These are required not only for postural control and movement but also to confer stability at the hip. It is called a ball and socket joint which permits movement of the legs in three directions — forwards and backwards (extension/flexion); inwards and outwards (adduction /abduction); and inward twist and outward twist (internal and external rotation).

The 3rd easy movement is an inward/outward rotating movement that corrects the misaligned tilt of the hips when done correctly. Gravity is once again your friend to assist in the corrections you are making.

The left and right hips move independently of each other. If one hip is tilted more forward than the other it can cause an elevation of the hip and then leads to offsets in the spine.

This exercise is done one leg at a time, so you can concentrate on this rotating action. Gravity works in concert with the rotational movement, so each hip can be gently guided to line up with the other hip utilizing the floor as reference.

Movement #4: Another correction for the hips.

Two or more corrective exercises are important for stabilizing the hip joint. Have you ever been told that one of your legs is shorter than the other? Have you noticed that you're constantly bearing more weight on one leg? Well then, it's very likely due to hip elevation. Exercise #3 corrects the pelvic tilt differences on the left and right sides. Exercise #4 is about correcting hip elevation so that the pelvic girdle is level. Gravity is our friend again as the pelvis sits on the floor to help with the leveling action.

I am going to repeat myself again because I care about you!

It is my desire to teach you a way to reduce pain naturally without drugs or surgery. You have the power within you to do this and only YOU can, because it takes willingness to learn how and then practice what you are taught. These **4 Easy Movements** can be done in less than 10 minutes. When they are done morning and night the magic happens—naturally.

I have been a part of the fitness industry for over 45 years. My trainings, especially as a Medical Exercise Specialist and Symmetry Practitioner, have taught me that poor posture is the foundational cause of most physical pain and many health issues. I am also a firm believer that all neuromotor abilities need to be addressed in fitness programming: Balance, Coordination, Flexibility and Strength (functional, endurance and power). I am excited about my program **Body Re-Design by Jacque** which combines Symmetry with all the wonderful trainings I have had throughout my career.

The beauty of **Body Re-Design** is that as your body heals, (becoming functionally stronger with better coordination and flexibility), the work of other practitioners available (i.e. acupuncture, chiropractic, massage etc.) can take you to new levels of optimal health. The healing that occurs affects all aspects of daily living. It is not only the physical body that becomes healthier, more energetic and productive, but also the mind and spirit as well.

May you be blessed and pain free.

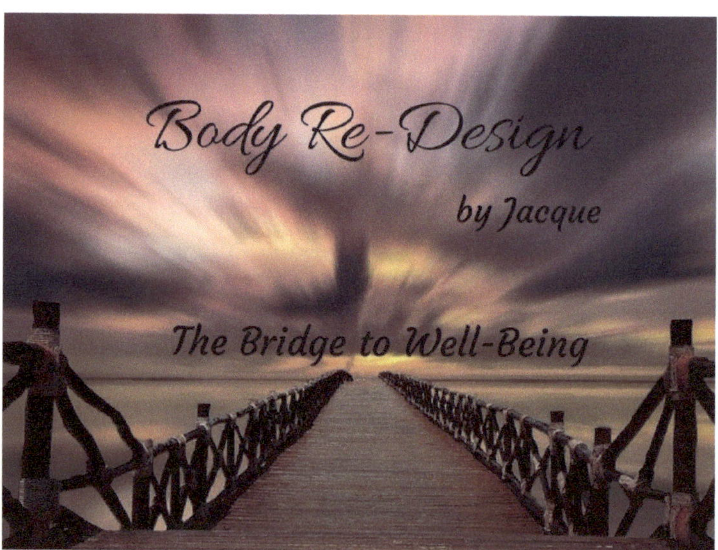

30 Intentions in 30 Days

Suggested Intentions

For A Healthier You

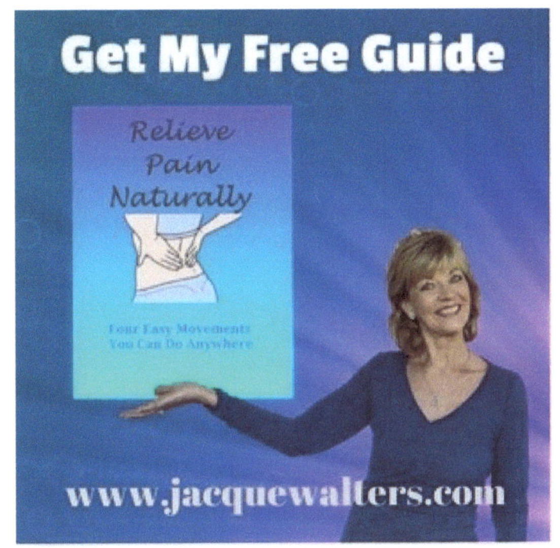

Intention #1

Give Symmetry a try. Do you have 8 minutes?

While talking on the phone, put the speaker option on and do the Four Easy Movements.

Did you download my free guide and watch the video?

(Yes, I know! You will get emails from me. But my main goal is information, not obligation. Remember you can always unsubscribe to my newsletters. The guide and video are still yours.)

Before doing the first movement, notice how your body is feeling. Is your neck stiff or sore? Does your back hurt? Do you feel pain in your hips? How are your knees feeling? (Write how you feel here.)

____

____

____

As you begin to settle into the first position, what areas of your body feel tight? If your back is extra tight, try placing a folded mat or pillow under your upper back and head. (Take note and then write them here after you have completed this "non-movement" exercise.)

____

____

____

____

Use the rest of this page to journal how each of the movements felt before and then after you completed them.

____

____

____

____

____

____

____

____

____

____

____

____

____

Intention #2

Throughout the day take as many extra steps as you can. The walking monitors are the "in thing" right now. Maybe consider getting one (if you don't have one) to see how many steps you do take each day.

- Take the stairs not the elevator.
- Park at a distance from the grocery store and appointments you may have and your work.
- At work do inconvenient walking. Go talk to a colleague instead of calling or emailing.
- Stand up often to drink water or go to the copying machine or file cabinet.
- During your break walk instead of sit.
- If your computer set up has the ability to allow you to stand, be sure to move around and not just stand in one place.
- Get up and move as often as possible just to move.
- If you feel tight hips when you walk or exercise, try this Pinwheel Stretch for Increased Flexibility.
- When watching TV, remember to stand up while changing the channel rather than just sitting. During commercials, even if you can fast-forward them, get up and move around until your show begins again. (Does anyone remember when there were no remotes?)

Did you do inconvenient walking and moving around today? (Write down here what you did.)

____

____

____

Did you check out my video?

What other ideas did you think of to keep moving?

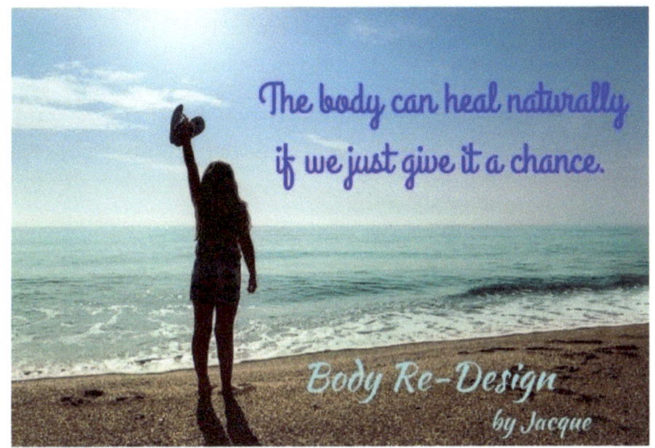

Intention #3

Write down 5 things you are grateful for. Read them through-out the day. Be sure to stand and walk around as you read them.

What are the five things you are grateful for? Take full deep breaths as you write each one.

1. ______________________________

____

2. ______________________________

____

3. ______________________________

____

4. ______________________________

____

5. ______________________________

____

How many times did you read them today? ______________

Write down what you did to move while you read them.

____

____

____

What other emotions came up while reading them?

____

____

____

____

Did you feel the gratitude in your both your mind and heart?
(Or any other area in the body?)

____

____

____

____

Journal how you felt after you read each one.

____

____

____

____

____

____

____

____

____

____

Intention #4

Take 3 minutes and do my version of the Nitric Oxide Dump.

Are you curious what that is?

Journal your experience.

____

____

____

____

____

____

____

____

____

____

____

____

____

____

____

____

Intention #5

Sometime today hold on to a counter, a railing, or a chair, and do 10 slow squats going only as low as your body allows. You can also open a door and hold the door knobs to squat.

How many squats did you do? ________________________________

(If you felt pain or discomfort in the knees then this intention is not for you.)

Did you do more than one set of 10?

____

Did you get inspired to do other movements?

____

____

____

Write down how this little exercise made you feel (both physically and emotionally) even though it only took about a minute.

____

____

____

____

____

____

____

____

Intention # 6

Today take a 5 to 10 minute gratitude walk. If possible do this in nature. If you live in the city, go to a park nearby. Focus on the scrubs, flowers

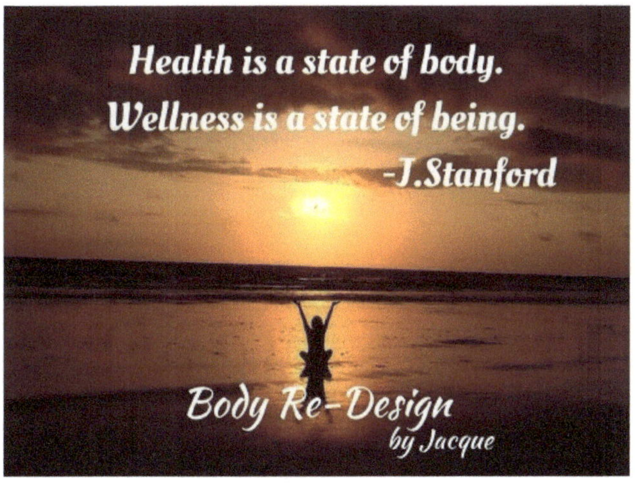

and trees. Take notice of birds flying among the trees, bees buzzing above the flowers, and butterflies flitting around the scrubs. Think about the 5 things you wrote down that you are grateful for. If you have foot pain or flat feet, check out this video about Easy Corrective Exercises for Over-Pronation.

How many times did your mind wander to thinking about what you needed to get done, or a problem you were trying to solve, or anything that was not in the present moment feeling gratitude.

____

Briefly write these wandering thoughts down.

____

____

____

____

____

____

Intention # 7

Set the alarm on your cell phone or computer to go off every hour (try this just for today). When it does, take five slow deep breaths while standing. Extend your arms forward and up as far as you can reach while inhaling deeply. Then open them up like you are holding a giant beach ball. As you exhale, lower your arms into the shape of a "W" and bring your elbows down as if you were putting them in your back pocket. I demonstrate this exercise in my video on How to Counteract the Negative Effects of Sitting.

Did you do "W" breathing?

____

Did you try any of the other exercises I demonstrate on my video?

____

Journal how you felt before and after.

____

____

____

____

____

____

____

____

____

Intention # 8

Check out my video <u>Water Infusion Ideas for Proper Hydration.</u> I talk about the wonderful health benefits infusing mint, lemon, and rosemary. Just for today, give it a try!

Did you give it a try?

____

How did it taste to you?

____

Did you drink more water because it tasted so good?

____

Write down other fruits and herbs that you might try.

____

____

____

____

____

____

____

____

____

____

Intention #9

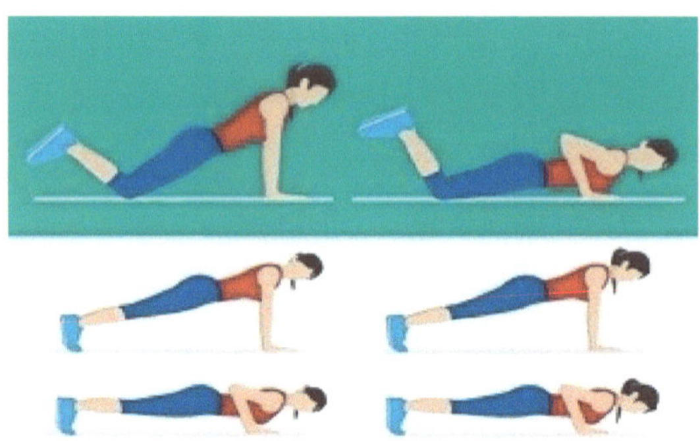

Do pushups with your hands on a wall or as shown in the picture.

Repeat 10 to 20 times.

 Go to Vecteezy.com for free photos.

How many push-ups did you do?

____

(If you felt pain or discomfort then this intention is not for you)

How did your body feel?

____

____

____

____

Were you inspired to do anything else? If so, write them here.

____

____

____

____

____

Intention #10

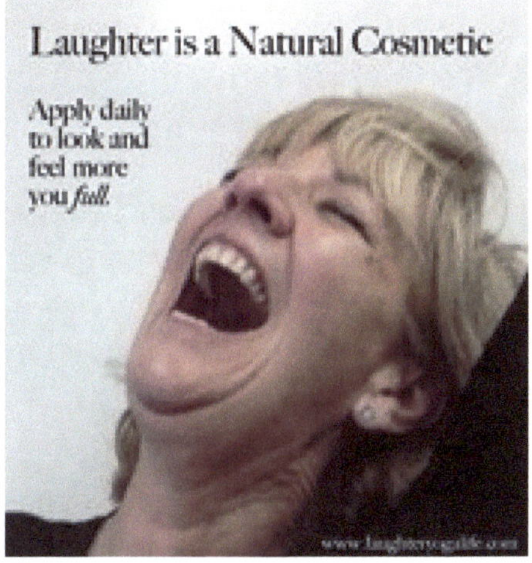

(Dr. William Fry, Stanford University) said that one minute of hardy laughter equals ten minutes on a row machine. There are many hilarious videos on YouTube. Do a quick search of babies giggling. It is nearly impossible to keep from laughing as you watch these little guys laugh. Watch my video Make Intentions Not Resolutions.

Did you make Intentions instead of Resolutions?

____

Did you watch a brief video of a baby laughing?
(I smile just thinking about how funny they are!)

____

Write down what your intentions are here.

____

____

____

____

____

____

Intention # 11

If you find that your neck muscles (back of the neck) are frequently tight and stiff, watch my video about an easy way to release those tight muscles.

Intention #12

Throughout the day, for a minute or two, become aware of how you are walking. Feel your feet as you take each step. Become aware of how your body is feeling as you "Center" yourself with this awareness. There is research that suggests that walking barefoot on the ground has many health benefits.

Intention #13

Take 2 ½ minutes to watch my video Over 90% of the Brain's Output is Used for Posture.

Did you release your tight neck muscles? _____________________

Did you walk barefoot on the ground? _____________________

Were you shocked by how much of the brain is used for posture?

____

Journal your thoughts here.

____

____

____

____

____

Intention #14

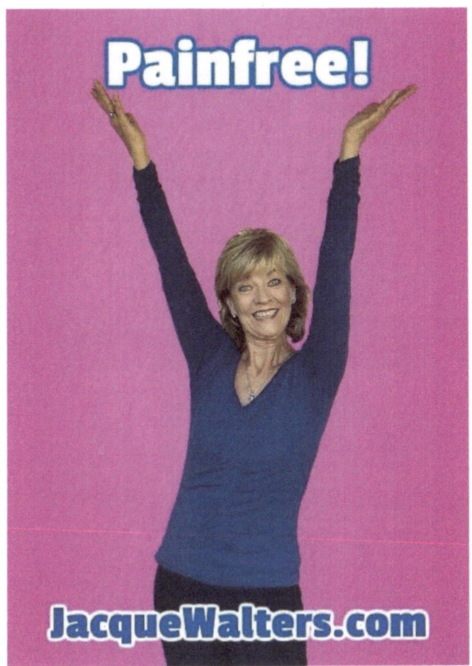

To strengthen your transverse abdominal muscle (your natural weight belt) take a deep breath and then pull your belly button to your spine and hold for 10 seconds (but don't hold your breath). Release and take deep belly breaths.

When driving practice this every time you come to a stop sign or stoplight. This is great to practice if you are in commuter traffic. You may want to put a sticker reminder on your steering wheel.

Remember to pull in and contract the abs every time you bend forward to protect your back. With practice this will happen automatically.

How many times did you practice this? _______________________

Did you notice any changes in your body? _______________________

Did you realize that your abs did not automatically pull in when you bent over? _______________________

Jot down your thoughts.

____

____

____

Intention #15

When feeling over-whelmed, take a step back and do something kind for yourself. Retreat to a quiet safe place where you can "just be" for 5 minutes. This would be a good

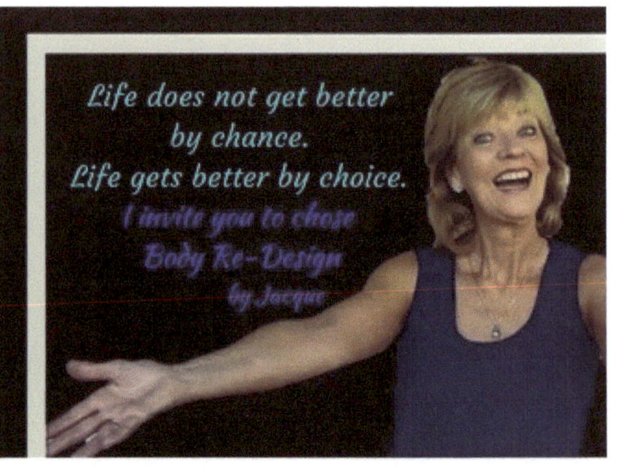

time to do the first exercise in the 4 Easy Movements. Breathe deeply and focus only on your breath. Never ever say anything negative to yourself about yourself, AND especially never put yourself down to others. You deserve to be loved and that love begins with self-love.

Write down one of your best qualities.

____

____

____

____

Do you have others that you can think of?

____

____

____

____

____

Use this space to write down your qualities and the pride you feel. Rewrite a negative thought into a positive thought. (i.e.: "I feel pressured with not enough time"—to—"I have all the time I need to get done what needs to be done.")

Intention #16

Watch my video interviewing a fellow fitness professional <u>A Special Treat for Happy Feet.</u> Learn about the many health benefits. Kick off your shoes and socks and join us!

Did you see and feel the difference in your feet?

____

____

____

____

How did you feel when you got up and moved around?

____

____

____

____

____

____

Do you think this is an easy 1-2 minute routine to add each morning or night?

____

Jot down your thoughts.

____

____

____

Intention #17

 If you have any type of cardio fitness equipment, perform 4-10 minutes of aerobic exercise. Change your pace throughout the minutes. Go faster or change the resistance for 15 to 20 seconds pushing to a higher intensity. Then return to a slower steady pace. Do this for 4-8 rounds. Just do what you can. Every little bit helps.

What equipment did you use?

____

____

____

How many seconds could you go at a higher intensity?

____

____

How many rounds of higher intensity were you able to do?

____

____

How did you feel after doing this type of cardio exercise?

____

____

____

____

____

Intention #18

It has been suggested that we should brush our teeth for 2 minutes. While brushing your teeth do 2 sets of 10 squats or a wall sit (also called an air bench sit) for as long as you can. You could also balance on one leg for one minute and repeat on the other side.

Which exercise did you choose?

____

Did you do more than one?

____

How did your body feel after you performed the exercise?

____

____

Intention #19

If you are having some hip or groin pain, watch [Psoas Stretch to Relieve Hip and Groin Pain.](#)

Did you watch the video? _________________________________

Did you give the release a try? _____________________________

How did you feel after the release?

____

____

____

____

____

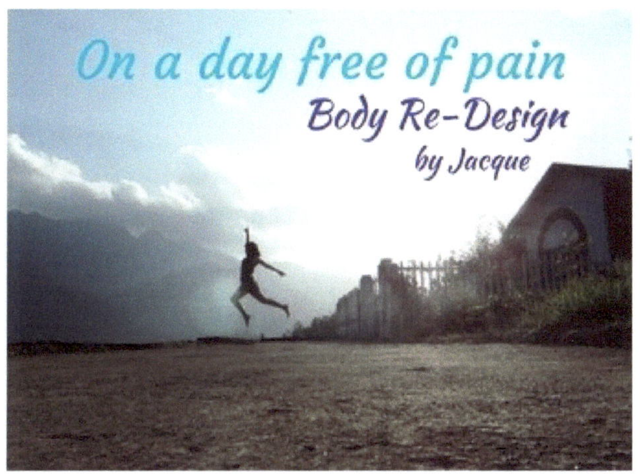

Intention #20

Ladies, if you wear mascara, while applying lean forward resting your hips on the counter and do leg extensions to wake up your "butt" muscles. (Lift one leg straight back behind you with your foot flexed and leg lengthened as you lift 20 times. Then repeat with the other leg. Be careful to maintain a neutral spine, not arching the low back.)

Men, you can do the same thing while shaving.

How many repetitions could you do before you felt a burn? (More than 20?)

____

Did you do more than one set?

____

What other creative exercise could you do?

____

____

____

____

____

Intention #21

Add essential oils to wet paper towels or non-toxic baby wipes. Place in a small zip lock bag. I use thyme, peppermint, and eucalyptus. I just put a drop or 2 on each towel. Then when running errands like grocery shopping I take one out and wipe my hands, the steering wheel, keys and gear shift after shopping before I start driving. When flying I wipe down everything I touch. This includes the seat belt, arm rests, any buttons and even the TV if there is one. Then I hold another near my nose as

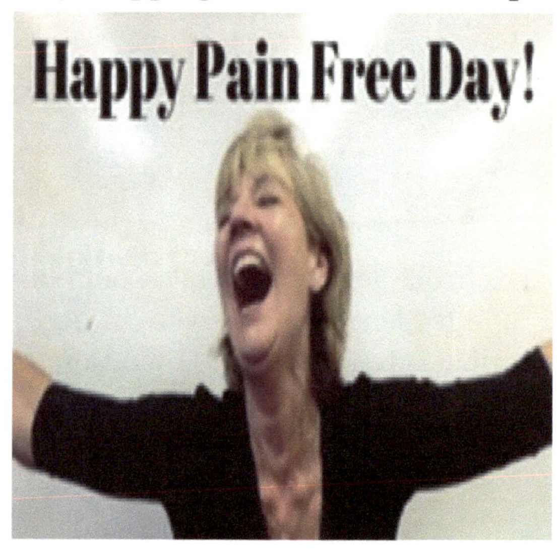

people are boarding and walk by me. I fly a lot and never catch any "bugs" on my flights. (Do not use these particular oils around small children, especially babies, or if you are pregnant as there are contraindications).

What are your favorite essential oils?

____

____

Can you come up with other combinations?
Write your ideas here.

____

____

Intention #22

While waiting for your coffee to brew or water for tea to boil, stand and do side lateral raises. Squeeze your shoulder blades without shrugging your shoulders. Start with your arms at your sides then slowly raise them toward the ceiling while inhaling. When they are shoulder height, turn the palms upward and continue raising your arms as high as you can comfortably. Exhale as you lower them. Repeat 2 sets of 10 reps. This exercise is helpful in correcting torso rotation and spinal offsets.

How did this exercise feel?

____

____

____

____

Could you do more than I suggested?

____

____

What other things could you do?

____

____

____

____

____

____

____

Intention #23

While flossing your teeth, stand on one leg and perform 20 ankle circles each direction on the non-weight bearing leg. Repeat on the other side. You can use the bath counter to lean against for support.

Then squeeze and release the "butt" muscles. Do 2 sets of 20 squeezes.

How did these exercises feel?

____

____

____

____

Could you do more than I suggested?

____

____

What other things could you do?

____

____

____

____

____

____

____

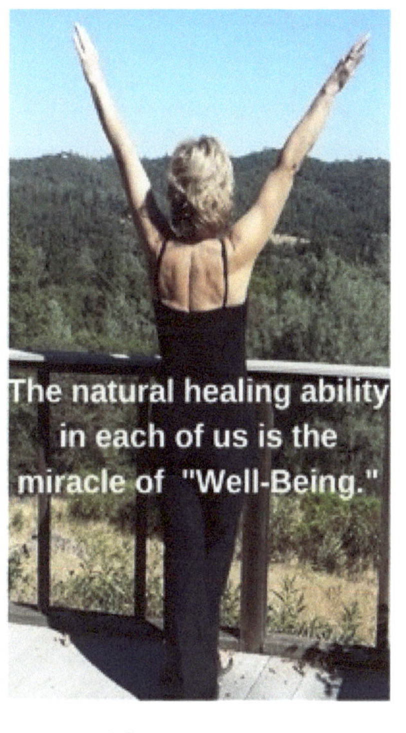

Intention # 24

I watch webinars on my computer and iPad while sitting on a Swiss ball. Here are some ideas and ways to move while watching.

• Perform bouncing squats. Gently bounce and hold in a squat position just above the ball for 1-2 seconds then bounce (only one time) and repeat. Do for 30 seconds to a minute.

• Do a modified side plank with your hand on the desk. Do 15 seconds to 1 minute on both sides.

• Hip abduction exercises 10-20x each leg (While standing on one leg, lift your other leg out to the side. Then repeat with the other leg.)

• Desk push-ups: (See push up pictures Intention #9). This time place your hands on your desk while pushing.

Which exercises did you do?

____

____

____

How many repetitions did you get in before having to jot down any notes you were taking from the webinar?

____

Did you do more than one set of an exercise?

Write down how creative you were.

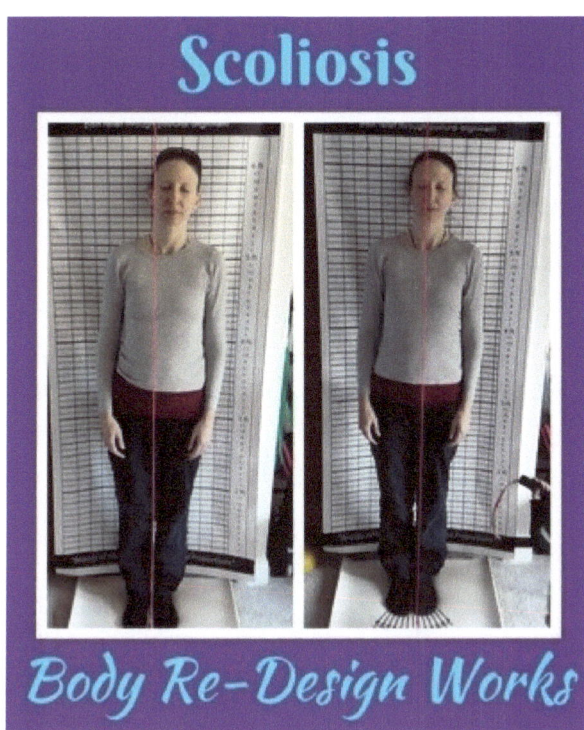

Intention #25

Do this simple "Howl at the Moon" stretch to relieve tightness in your neck.

Check out these before and after shots (scoliosis)! Proof that Body Re-Design works! How could Body Re-Design help you?

Jot down how you felt before and then after you did the "Howl at the Moon" stretch.

____

____

____

____

____

How could you fit this stretch into your day?

____

____

____

____

Intention #26

Think about something nice that you do for others. Do this exercise as if a good friend were talking about you. This is subtly different than your qualities of #5. (i.e. She always smiles easily at others, even strangers.) See if you (your friend) can come up with 10.

Then repeat your nice statements about yourself while doing the **Sit to Stand Exercise**: From a sitting position in your chair, stand and slowly lower back down to sitting. Repeat this for every one of your 10 positive statements.

1. ____

2. ____

3. ____

4. ____

5. ____

6. ____

7. ____

8. ____

9. ____

10. ____

How do feel physically and emotionally after incorporating these positive affirmations into your movement?

____

____

Intention #27

Get up and turn on your favorite lively song and dance your heart out for just a few minutes!

What physical changes did you feel?

____

____

What emotional changes did you feel?

____

____

Intention #28

Today look for one thing that you believe is a miracle. This could be anything like a cloud that looks like an animal or angel. (My grandson can find an alligator in every cloud). Or maybe a hummingbird that comes to visit you at your kitchen window. I believe miracles are everywhere. For me, waking up pain free is my biggest miracle.

Write down the first miracle that came to mind.

____

____

____

Can you thinks of any other miracles?

____

____

____

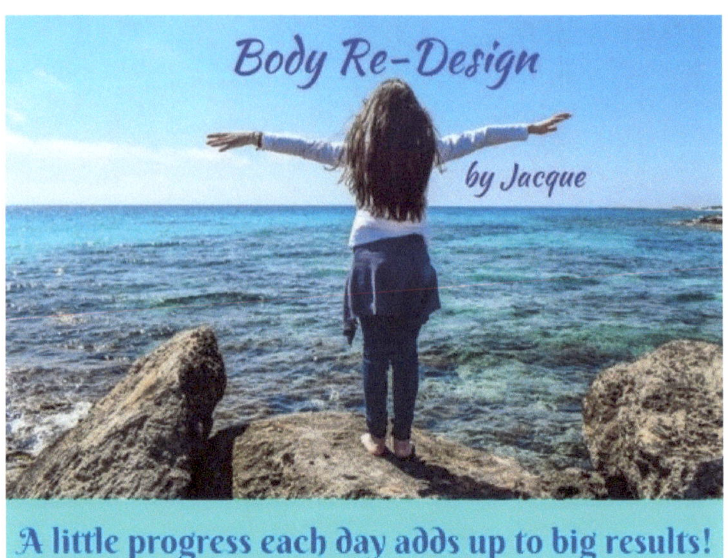

Intention #29

When washing or rinsing dishes do heel raises. Then stand on a wedge (a 3-ring binder works) to stretch them out.

How many were you able to do before you felt a burn?

____

Did you do more than one set of repetitions?

____

Can you think of other exercises that you can do while washing dishes (i.e. rocking your hips side to side)?

____

____

____

____

____

Intention #30

Watch my video on the [Benefits of Apple Cider Vinegar](). If you already drink this everyday as I do, I invite you to watch my video in order to be reminded of what a good thing you are doing for your body. Then pat yourself on the back.

How did you like learning about or being reminded about the many benefits?

____

____

____

What was your favorite benefit?

____

____

What other daily health benefits can you think of that only take seconds to do? (Take a deep breath before you write)

____

____

____

____

____

____

____

(Now blink your eyes several times to moisten and relieve pressure.)

Final Reflections

What intentions did you find the most beneficial? Why?

____

____

____

____

____

____

____

What was the most important thing you have learned from your journaling in this workbook? Why?

____

____

____

____

____

____

____

____

By now I bet you have come up with more ideas of your own. Write them down below. Then, of course, do them.

Thank you for working through these

30 Intentions in 30 Days.

I sincerely hope you found the suggested intentions useful. If you liked my ideas, please subscribe to my YouTube channel, www.youtube.com/jacquewalters for all my fit tips and also follow me on Facebook: https://www.facebook.com/JacqueBodyRedesign/.

I offer a free mini-consultation to answer any questions you may have about fitness or postural re-alignment programming. You can call or text me at 408-489-2011. These consults are all about information with no obligation.

http://www.jacquewalters.com/services/

I am also available for speaking engagements, presentations, and workshops (virtual and in-person).

I am here for you.

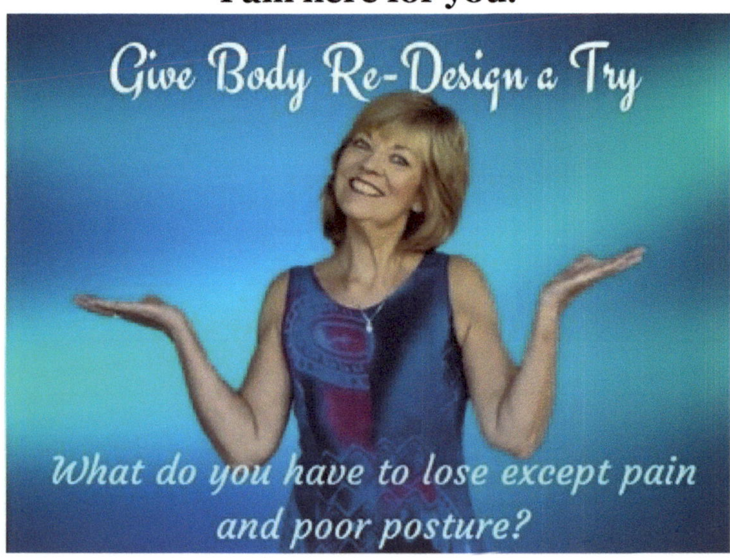

Please feel free to share this book with anyone that you think would enjoy these ideas or want to begin to re-align the body for pain relief and optimal health.

Link Addresses

The quickest and easiest way to watch Jacque's videos is to go directly to her YouTube channel! Here you can scroll through and watch any of her videos. Don't forget to subscribe so you don't miss out on her future video tips!

www.youtube.com/jacquewalters

Here is a list of direct links.

4 Easy Movements: http://www.jacquewalters.com/4emoptin/
Sitting Too Much: http://www.jacquewalters.com/2017/09/13/are-you-sitting-too-much/
90% of Brain's Output: https://youtu.be/AiUXWbriHig
Pinwheel Stretch for Flexibility: https://youtu.be/EBHBMQ7Z7O0
Nitric Oxide Dump: https://youtu.be/QLR-CgrvfRc
Over-Pronation: https://youtu.be/-DDHoDI4EzQ
Negative Effects of Sitting: https://youtu.be/tiCVNdBsW9g
Water Infusion: https://youtu.be/JAOSL2B3pM4
Intentions not Resolutions: https://youtu.be/M2m6tQzmuxQ
Neck Release: https://youtu.be/WTJNbtW018I
Bare Feet Treat: https://youtu.be/fUtBbzWkNhg
Psoas Stretch: https://youtu.be/7Oa5ZKmby0U
Howl at the Moon Neck Stretch: https://youtu.be/jd3yxgYhz3I
Apple Cider Vinegar: https://youtu.be/8Crx_UO5dNQ

I want to acknowledge and thank www.pixabay.com for all their beautiful free pictures.

And, of course, don't miss out on all the great tips on her website and check out her Mountain Retreat page while you're there!
www.JacqueWalters.com

Follow Jacque on Facebook for even more pain-free and healthy living tips!
Fb.me/JacqueBodyRedesign

ABOUT THE AUTHOR

Jacque graduated from the University of Wisconsin as a Bio-psychological Development Specialist. This independent degree combines studies in Physical Education, Physiology, Adapted Physical Education, Exercise Science, Psychology, Rehabilitation Psychology and Communication. She is certified as a personal trainer through the National Academy of Sports Medicine (NASM), and as a health and fitness specialist through the American College of Sports Medicine (ACSM), American Council on Exercise (ACE), Aquatic Exercise Association (AEA.) and the Kenneth Cooper Institute for Aerobics Research. She completed a certification as a Medical Exercise Specialist through the American Academy of Heath, Fitness and Rehabilitation Professionals (AAHFRP) and as a Postural Therapist "Symmetry" Practitioner.

It is Jacque's desire to assist individuals to a higher level of health and well-being through her personalized fitness programs. She also provides workshops and events to inspire, motivate, and educate.

Learn more at www.JacqueWalters.com

www.ingramcontent.com/pod-product-compliance
Lightning Source LLC
Chambersburg PA
CBHW040237240726
48664CB00001B/161